NOTICES

With the rapid advancements in technology and Knowledge, best practice in this field is constantly changing. Therefore it's preferable to always rely on their own experience and knowledge in evaluating and using any information in form of methods, experiments or anyways per say described herein. At every point in using information from this book take all appropriate safety precautions for self and other parties.

With respect to any drug or pharmaceutical products mentioned or described related to anything herein, readers are advised to check the most current information provided on package inserts, material safety data sheet (MSDS), by supplier or by the manufacturer.

If using this book as a practitioner. It is advisable to rely on own experience and knowledge of their patients, to make diagnoses and accordingly tailor the best treatment/dosage for the patient. Repeating again to take all appropriate safety precautions.

As a matter of products liability neither the Publisher nor the authors/editors takes responsibility for any injury and/or damage to persons or property, on the use or operation of any instructions, ideas, methods or products contained in the book herein.

ABOUT THE AUTHOR

It took me almost 3 years and 8 months to publish my first book. It's my sincere effort in distilling the essential information from each of selected fields and creating readable and authoritative notes published in the form of book. I did my graduation in year 2005. My main subjects were microbiology ad biochemistry. My career started in year 2005. I continued with my studies and also my practice after marriage. In year 2013 I left Sant Gajanan Maharaj Rural hospital and Research Centre, where I was working as a lecturer and medical laboratory technician. I completed my post-graduation in advance medical laboratory technology in year 2013. In year 2015 undergone ISO 15189:2012 – internal audit course by DAC in Dubai. And I am working as quality manager and lab Technologist in Dubai. ISO 15189:2012 is a standard for medical laboratories. In year 2019 I did my post-graduation in Total quality management from Mumbai, India.

PREFACE

This book strives to provide the basic fundamental background knowledge by which a learner can be introduced to these practices and to serve as a resource for laboratory personnel and building up of a concept. These are the microbes of various morphological features. They are responsible for variety of diseases. They may cause trivial infections such as amoebiasis, ringworm and influenza to dreaded and fatal disease like cerebral malaria, cerebral cryptococosis to AIDS.

Study of these microbes helps in pinpointing etiologic agent of infectious disease as well as for epidemiology and vaccine preparation.

The book/notes can be considered as a source of information/ academic performance for students, and personnel's in the discipline of clinical pathology and laboratory medicine, and for physicians and laboratory practitioners. Color illustrations have been used throughout the book to accurately, realistically depict to provide clear image of subject.

OBJECTIVES of the book:

To develop the skill of laboratory diagnosis of various parasites, Pathogenic fungi and viruses

ACKNOWLEDGMENTS

I am grateful to my husband and my son who were always with me every moment in thick and thin of life while writing notes. I would take this opportunity to thank each one in my family for their timely support and being available whenever I needed them. Also to all of my students and colleagues who have contributed enormously to the development of my knowledge in the use of laboratories for diagnosis and patient management. I am grateful for their stimulus provided to my professional growth and ultimately to come up with a book. They have made this endeavor a happy one. I am especially grateful for the mentorship and encouragement provided in my career by Dr. Yashwant Chavan and Mr. Sirish Ganacharya. My sincere gratitude to student and staff of "Sant Gajanan Maharaj Rural Hospital & Research Centre", Mahagaon Maharashtra.

Upon the completion of the first edition, I humbly thank all the individuals who have played roles in making it possible. Since thank giving list seems to be endless, It is not possible to name all of the individuals who have contributed to this book. To those mentioned here and to those not explicitly named, I humbly thank you for your prodigious efforts and support.

TABLE OF CONTENT

Introduction of virology	4
General properties of viruses	4
Structure of virus	5
Classification of viruses	7
Laboratory diagnosis of viral infections	10
Specimen collection	10
Transportation and Storage of Specimen	11
Laboratory diagnosis	11
Cultivation of virus	11
Bacteriophage and its significance	16
Life Cycle of Bacteriophage and Replication of Viruses	17
A. Lytic Cycle	17
B. Lysogenic Cycle	19
Morphology, Pathogenicity and Laboratory Diagnosis of Hepatitis Viruses	20
Hepatitis A virus	20
Hepatitis B virus	22
Hepatitis C virus	24
Hepatitis D virus	26
Hepatitis E virus	28
Morphology, Pathogenicity and Laboratory Diagnosis of HIV / AIDS Virus.	29
Oncogenic viruses	34
REFERENCES	36

INTRODUCTION OF VIROLOGY

Terminology

Virology	The study of viruses is called as virology.
Virion	Infectious virus particle
Capsid	Protein shell which surrounds and protects the genome. It is built up of multiple (identical) protein sub-units called capsomers. Capsids are either icosahedral or tubular in shape.
Nucleocapsid	Genome + capsid.
Envelope	Lipoprotein membrane which surrounds some viruses, derived from the plasma membrane of the host cell.
Glycoproteins	Proteins found in the envelope of the virion; usually glycosylated.

HISTORY:

Year	Scientist name	Contribution
1897	Beijerinck	Discovered and coined the term virus.
1935	Wendell Stanley	Discovered that viruses are composed of nucleic acids, protein and lipids.

General properties of viruses

The term virus is derived from Latin word-"virus" means poison.

General Properties of Viruses
- Viruses are "living" in living thing and non-living in non-living things.
- They contain only one type of nucleic acid, either DNA or RNA but never both.
- They are obligate intracellular parasites.
- They lack the enzymes necessary for metabolic activities like protein and nucleic acid synthesis.
- They are dependent for replication on host cells.
- They multiply by a complex process.
- Viruses are much smaller than bacteria. They are too small to be seen under the light microscope.
- They are sensitive to interferon.
- The medical importance of viruses lies in their ability to cause a very large number of human diseases, from minor ailments like common cold to terrifying diseases like rabies and AIDS.

Viruses are living in the 'living' and non-living in non-living things.

Viruses are obligate intracellular parasites. They lack the enzymes necessary for metabolic activities like protein and nucleic acid synthesis. They are dependent for replication on host cells. They multiply by a complex process. They are unaffected by antibacterial antibiotics. Therefore they can survive only in living host but not on non living things.

Viruses Size:

Viruses Size	20 nm to 300 nm
Largest viruses	Poxviruses
Smallest DNA viruses	parvoviruses
Smallest RNA viruses	Picornavirus

Shape:
  i. Rabies virus is bullet shaped.
  ii. Pox virus is brick shaped.
  iii. Polio virus is spherical shape.

Structure of virus-

The typical structure of virus contains the following:
1. Central core consist of nucleic acid (RNA or DNA)
2. Protein coat around central core is called capsid.
3. Subunit of capsid is known as capsomers.
4. Envelope.
5. Protein subunits on surface of envelope known as peplomers.

1. **Nucleic acid** -contains 3-400 genes

Deoxyribonucleic Acid (DNA) -unique features
  - Single and/or double stranded
  - Glycosylated and/or Gaps present in double stranded molecule
  - Circular or linear
  - Bound to protein molecules
  - Unique purine and/or pyrimidine bases present
  - Ribonucleotides present

Ribonucleic Acid (RNA)
  - Single or double stranded
  - Segmented or unsegment
  - Bound protein molecules
  - Unique purine and/or pyrimidine bases present

2. Capsid -The capsid accounts for most of the virion mass. It is the protein coat of the virus. It is a complex and highly organized structure which gives form to the virus. Subunits of protomeres aggregate to form capsomers which in turn aggregate to form the capsid of the virus. There are 2 forms of symmetry:

Capsid Symmetry	Arrangement of capsid	Example	Presentation
Icosahedral	Capsomers arranged in 20 triangles	Polioviruses	Fig.1
Helical	Arranged in a hollow coil that appears rod-shaped	Rabies virus	Fig.2

Functions of the viral capsid:
1. Protect the genetic material mediate attachment
2. Site of receptors
3. Serve as antigenic determinants
4. Induce antibody production
5. Determinants of type specificity
6. Provide the structural symmetry of the virus

   3. **Envelope** -this is an amorphous structure composed of glycoproteins (peplomers) that appear as spikes which lies to the outside of the capsid. It is acquired through budding from the host's cell membrane in the course of maturation. It is more sensitive to heat, detergents.

Functions:
1. Site of receptors - attach to host cell receptors & membrane fusion
2. Antigenic determinants
3. Stimulate antibody production
4. Determinants of type specificity

4. Spikes. These are glycoprotein projections which have enzymatic and/or adsorption and/or hemagglutination activity. They arise from the envelope and are highly antigenic.

Classification of viruses

Viruses are mainly classified by Genome structure, nucleic acid type, capsid and depending on mRNA production.

1. ICTV classification-
The International Committee on Taxonomy of Viruses began to classification of viruses early in the 1970s. The system shares viral classifications at the level of order and continues as follows, with the taxon suffixes given in italics:

Order (-*virales*)
Family (-*viridae*)
Subfamily (-*virinae*)
Genus (-*virus*)
Species
Species names usually take the form of [Disease] virus, significantly for higher plants and animals.

2. Virus classification by genome structure and core:
The type of genetic material and its structure are used to classify the virus core structures.
Major groups of DNA virus:-

Virus	Size	Core Genome	Envelope	Cause
Adeno	70-90 nm	Double stranded DNA	Absent	Acute respiratory disease, pharyngitis and conjunctivitis
Herpes	100-200 nm	Double stranded DNA	Sensitive envelope	Versical skin lesions, encephalitis, chickenpox, etc…
Hepadnavirus	42 nm	Circular DNA and are partially double stranded	Absent	Acute and chronic hepatitis. Persistent infections are associated with a high risk of developing liver cancer.
Pox virus	230-300 X 200-250 nm, Large, brick shaped or Ovoid virus	Double stranded DNA	Lipid containing Envelope	Tend to produce skin lesions

Papovavirus	40-50nm			Causes human warts, papillomata of rabbits & polyma of mice. It produces chronic infection in hosts.
Parvoviruses	20 nm	Single stranded DNA	Absent	Causes gastroenteritis while other are associated with hemolytic disease.

Major groups of RNA virus:-

Virus	Size	Core Genome	Envelope	Cause
Retrovirus	90-120 nm in diameter	Single stranded RNA		Family contains many tumor producing viruses such as Sarcoma Virus. HIV (Human immunodeficiency virus which is the causative agent for AIDS (Acquired immunodeficiency syndrome) belong to this family.
Rhabdovirus	50-95 X 130-390 nm	Single stranded RNA	Present	Examples are Rabies Virus, vesicular stomatitis virus etc… Rabies virus causes infection of central nervous system.
Orthomyxovirus	80-120 nm	Single stranded RNA		They may cause influenza etc… Examples are influenza virus type A, B and C, etc…
Paramyxoviruses	150-300 nm	Single stranded RNA	Present	Causes respiratory infections, bad cold, measles, mumps, etc… Examples are parainfluenza virus 1 to 4, measles virus.
Tangovirus	40-70 nm	Single stranded RNA	Present	The virus causes meningoencephalitis, lymphadenopathy, bleeding and purpuric rashes, yellow fever, etc. Examples are- yellow fever, and dengue viruses.
Arenavirus	85-12 nm	Single stranded RNA	Present	They cause benign meningitis and encephalitis e.g. lymphocytic choriomeningitis virus, etc…
Reovirus	60-80 nm	Double stranded RNA	Present	Cause gastroenteritis.

Picornavirus	20-30 nm	Single stranded RNA		Examples- rhinoviruses (causing common cold) and enterovirus (causing polio)
Coronavirus	80-130 nm	Single stranded RNA	Present	Causes acute respiratory infection, mouse hepatitis etc... Examples- human murine and avian virus.

3. Virus classified by capsid structure:

Viruses can also be classified based on the design of their capsids.

Capsid classification	Examples
Naked icosahedral	Hepatitis A virus, polioviruses
Enveloped icosahedral	Epstein- Barr virus, herpes simplex virus, rubella virus, yellow fever virus, HIV-1
Naked helical	Tobacco mosaic virus
Enveloped helical	Influenza viruses, mumps virus, rabies virus
Complex capsid structures	Herpes viruses, smallpox virus, hepatitis B virus, T4 bacteriophage

4. Baltimore classification

The most commonly used was developed by biologist David Baltimore in the early 1970's. It is based on the mRNA production during the replicative cycle of the virus, in addition to other criteria's.

Group	Characteristics	Mode of mRNA production	Example
I.	Double stranded DNA	mRNA is transcribed directly from the DNA template	Herpes virus
II.	Single stranded DNA	DNA is converted to double stranded form before RNA is transcribed	Parvovirus
III.	Double stranded RNA	mRNA is transcribed form the RNA genome	Rotavirus
IV.	Single stranded RNA (+)	Genome function as mRNA	Picornavirus
V.	Single stranded RNA (-)	mRNA is transcribed form the RNA genome	Rabies virus
VI.	Single stranded RNA with reverse transcriptase	Reverse transcriptase makes DNA from the RNA genome. DNA is then incorporated in the genome; mRNA is transcribed from the incorporated DNA	HIV
VII.	Double stranded DNA	The viral genome is double stranded	Hepatitis B

	with reverse transcriptase	DNA but viral DNA is replaced through an RNA intermediate, the RNA may serve directly as mRNA or as a template to make mRNA.	virus

5. Holmes classification:

According to Holmes system of binomial nomenclature, viruses are classified into 3 groups under one order, Virales. They are placed as follows:
- Group I: *Phaginae* (attacks bacteria)
- Group II: *Phytophaginae* (attacks plants)
- Group III: *Zoophaginae* (attacks animals)

6. LHT System of Virus Classification:

The LHT System of Virus Classification is based on-
- Chemical and physical characters like nucleic acid (DNA or RNA),
- Symmetry (Helical or Icosahedral or Complex),
- Presence of envelope,
- Diameter of capsid and
- Number of capsomers.

Laboratory diagnosis of viral infections

Specimen collection-

SYSTEM	SPECIMEN	REQUIRED
	For isolation	For direct examination
Respiratory	Throat swab, Throat washings, Aspirates	Nasopharyngeal aspirate
Central Nervous System	Feces, Blood, CSF	Brain biopsy, CSF
Cardio Vascular System	Feces, Muscular pustular scrapings, ulcer scrapings, throat swab	Vesicular/Pustular fluid, Ulcer scraping.
Eye	Conjunctival scraping and swab	Conjunctival scraping/Swabs
Liver	Blood	Serum
Congenital infections	Throat swab, product of conception	NIL

Transportation and Storage of Specimen

All the samples ought to be transported to laboratory in a very sterile, leak proof container. The samples should be transported as soon as possible.
- In case of fragile viruses for e.g. RSV virus inoculation of cell cultures at the bed facet has been counseled.
- Swabs ought to be placed in infective agent transport media swabs only.
- The specimens should be refrigerated at -70°C if they are to be stored for a very long time (weeks or months). When the delay is short (less than 24 hours) specimens are stored at 4°C temperature.

Laboratory diagnosis

I. Microscopy:
It includes
1. Detection of viral inclusion body by light microscopy
2. Detection of virus or viral agents by using electron microscope.

II. **Demonstration of virus antigen**

Direct detections of virus antigen can be done in cases where the antigen is abundant in the lesions. It is demonstrated by serological methods such as precipitate in gel or immune fluorescence. Counter immune electrophoresis, radio immune assay & Enzyme Linked immunosorbent assay have found wide application in diagnostic virology for the detection of viral antigens in clinical samples.

Molecular methods like polymerase chain Reaction (PCR), Real time polymerase reaction (RT-PCR), Nucleic acid. For sensitive and rapid detection of viral antigens methods used are Sequence based Amplification (NASBA), Transcription Mediated Amplification (TMA), etc

III. **Methods for Cultivation of Virus**

The primary purpose of virus cultivation is:
1. To isolate and determine/identify viruses in clinical samples.
2. To do research analysis on viral structure, replication, biology, genetics and effects on host cell.
3. To prepare viruses for vaccine production.

CULTIVATION OF VIRUS

Generally three strategical methods are employed for the virus cultivation.

1. Inoculation of virus into animals.
2. Inoculation of virus into embryonated eggs.
3. Tissue culture

1. Inoculation of Virus in Animals

Laboratory animals are widely used for routine cultivation of virus; they play an important role in studies of viral pathological processes. Live animals such as monkeys, mice, rabbits, guinea pigs, ferrets and Mice are the most widely employed animals in virology. The different routes of inoculation in mice are intracerebral, subcutaneous, intraperitoneal or intranasal. The animal is observed for signs of disease or visible lesions after the inoculation of virus suspension. The infected tissues by virus can be examined.

Advantages:
1. Animal inoculation could also be used as diagnostic procedural technique.
2. For identifying and isolating a virus from a clinical specimen.
3. Mice provide a reliable model for studying viral replication.
4. Insight into viral pathogenesis and host virus relation.
5. For the study of immune responses, epidemiology and oncogenesis.

Disadvantages:
1. Expensive (overprice) and difficulties in maintenance of animals.
2. Difficulty in choosing of animals for specific virus.
3. Some human viruses cannot be grown, or can be grown in animal but do not cause disease.
4. Mice are not preferred as models for vaccine development.
5. It will result in generation of escape mutants.
6. Issues related to animal welfare systems.

2. Inoculation of Virus into Embryonated eggs

Good pasture in 1931first used the embryonated hen's egg for the cultivation of virus.
The process of cultivation of viruses in embryonated eggs depends on the site of egg which is used for virus inoculation. The egg used for cultivation should be sterile and also the shell should be intact and healthy. A hole is drilled in the shell of the healthy embryonated egg carefully.Through this hole a viral suspension or suspected virus- containing tissue is injected into the fluid of the egg. Viral growth and multiplication in is indicated by the death of the embryo, by embryo cell damage, or by the formation of typical pocks or lesions on the egg membranes.

The various sites offered by an embryonated egg for the cultivation of viruses are-
- Chorioallantoic Membrane(CAM).
- Amniotic Cavity.
- Allantoic Cavity

- Yolk Sac.
- Embryo.
- Air Sac.

Procedure for inoculation in chick embryo-
1. For propagation of influenza virus, pathogen-free eggs are used 11-12 days after fertilization.
2. The egg is placed in front of a light source to locate a non-veined area of the allantoic cavity just below the air sac. This is marked with a pencil.
3. A hole is drilled at the top of the egg with a Dremel motorized tool after a small nick.
4. After all the eggs have been nicked and drilled, they are inoculated with virus using a tuberculin syringe – a 1 ml syringe fitted with a 1/2 inch, 27 gauge needle.
5. The needle passes through the chorioallantoic membrane and reaches to allantoic cavity where the virus is placed.
6. The two holes in the shell are sealed with melted paraffin, and the eggs are placed at 37°C for 48 hours.

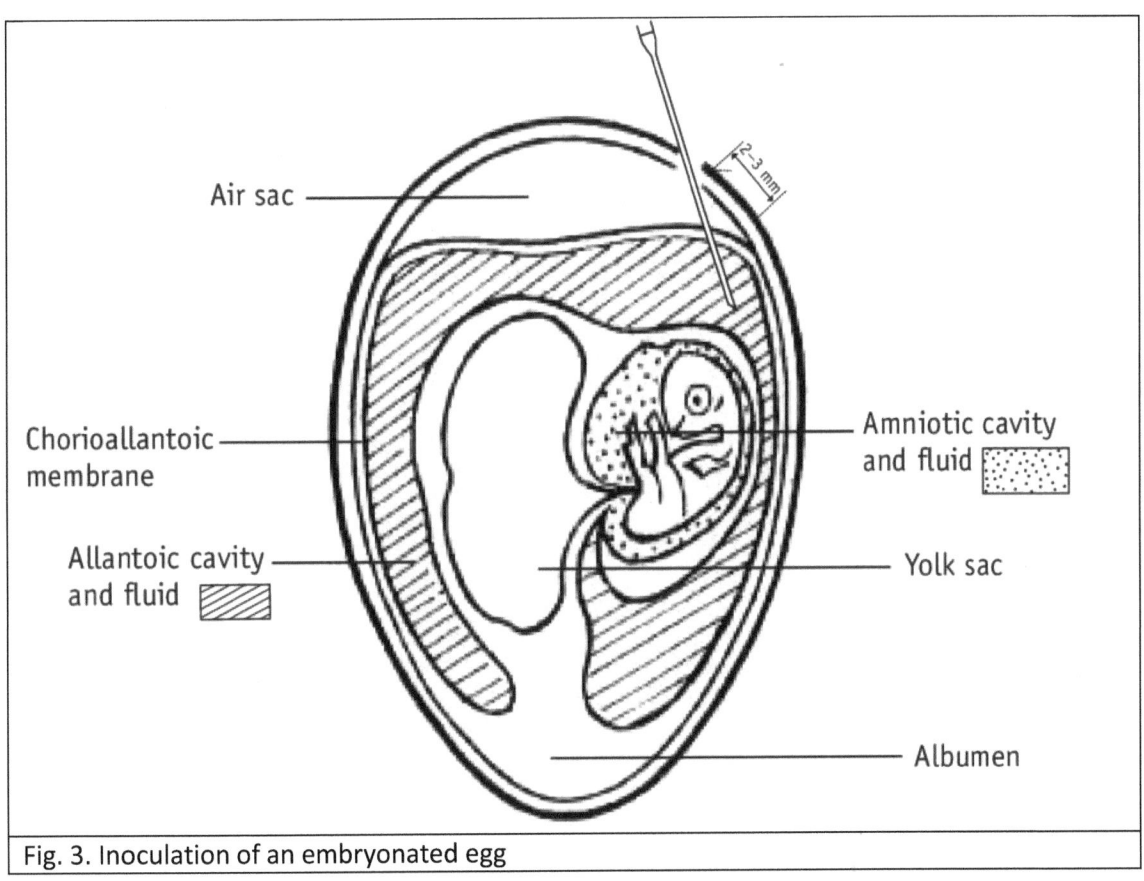

Fig. 3. Inoculation of an embryonated egg

Advantages:
- Widely used method for the isolation of virus and growth.
- Ideal substrate for the viral growth and replication.
- Isolation and cultivation of viruses.
- Cost effective and maintenance is much easier
- Less labor is needed.
- The embryonated eggs are readily available.
- Sterile and wide range of tissues and fluids
- They are sterile with respect to bacteria and viruses.
- There is no immune response of an embryonated eggs.
- Widely used method to grow virus for some vaccine production.

Disadvantages:
The site of immunization for varies with completely different virus. That is, every virus has completely different sites for his or her growth and replication.

3. Cell Culture (Tissue Culture)
There are three types of tissue culture;
- Organ culture,
- Explant culture and
- Cell culture.

A. Organ cultures are mainly done for highly specialized parasites of certain organs e.g. tracheal ring culture is done for isolation of coronavirus.

B. Explant culture is rarely done. It is a technique where living cells or tissues are removed from an embryo and developed outside the organism i.e. in vitro. This allows researchers to closely observe their investigation on developing tissues in ways that are not possible *in vivo*.

C. Cell culture is used for identification and cultivation of viruses. Cells are grown in vitro in a suitable growth medium under controlled conditions.

Advantages of cell culture
1. Relative ease, broad spectrum, cheaper and sensitivity

Disadvantage of cell culture
1. The process requires trained and experienced technicians.

2. State health laboratories and hospital laboratories are not involved in viruses studies in clinical work.
3. For identification of viruses, tissue or serum is sent to central laboratories.

4. Cultivation of plant viruses

There are some methods for Cultivation of plant viruses which can grow in whole plants such as plant tissue cultures, cultures of separated cells, or cultures of protoplasts, etc.

Procedure-

Leaves are rubbed with a mixture of viruses and an abrasive mechanically to inoculate with the desired virus. The abrasive breaks the cell wall of leaves. The plasma membrane is **exposed of and** comes directly in contact with virus. Once virus enters they control by adhering and easily infect the host cells.

Result- A localized necrotic lesion often develops due to the rapid death of cells in the infected area.

5. Cultivation of bacteriophages

Cultivated in either broth or agar cultures of young bacterial cells but for replication depends on living host.

IV. SEROLOGICAL DIAGNOSIS

The presence of an antibody to a virus only denotes that the person's immune system has been exposed to the viral antigen. Besides it could be a current infection by the virus, the antibody may have been formed by the following-
- A previous symptomatic / asymptomatic infection
- In response to cross reacting antigen and
- Vaccination

The level of the antibody remains nearly the same for the entire duration of current illness. However, to be an indicative of infection with the virus there should be a fourfold increase of antibody titer tested at an interval of 10 to 14 days.

There are varieties of methods available commercially in the market to diagnose viral infection by antibody detection. The choice of the method depends upon the sensitive of the test and intensity of immune response. Various tests available are ELISA, complement fixation test, neutralization, hemagglutination tests.

V. MOLECULAR TECHNIQUES

Various molecular technique which can be used in diagnosis of viral infections are-
1. Nucleic acid sequence based amplification (NASBA)
2. Transcription mediated amplification
3. Polymerase chain reaction
4. Real time polymerase chain reaction

The advantages of molecular techniques are that, they are rapid and are highly sensitive& specific.
The only disadvantage is that it requires technical expertise and is resource intensive.

Bacteriophage and its significance:

1. Introduction to Bacteriophage: Bacteriophage (Greek phage is—to eat; bacteriophage, bacteria-cater) are viruses that infect and parasitize bacteria. They cause lysis of bacteria. They are abbreviated as phages.

2. History: Frederick Twart (1915) and Felix d'Herelle (1917) observed an invisible minute parasite of bacteria that caused lysis of the culture of dysentery bacilli (Sh. shiga) and named it bacteriophage.

3. Habitat: Phages occur widely in association with bacteria in the environment (feces, sewages).

4. General Characteristics: Bacteriophages are highly host specific and, on the basis of phage, typing of bacteria is done.

5. Morphology of Bacteriophage:
The phages are tadpole-shaped and have a head and tail:

1. Head: It is hexagonal and contains a tightly packed core of nuclei acid (double-stranded DNA) covered by a protein coat (capsid). The head of phage T_4 measures 65nm in diameter. It is approx. 100 nm long.	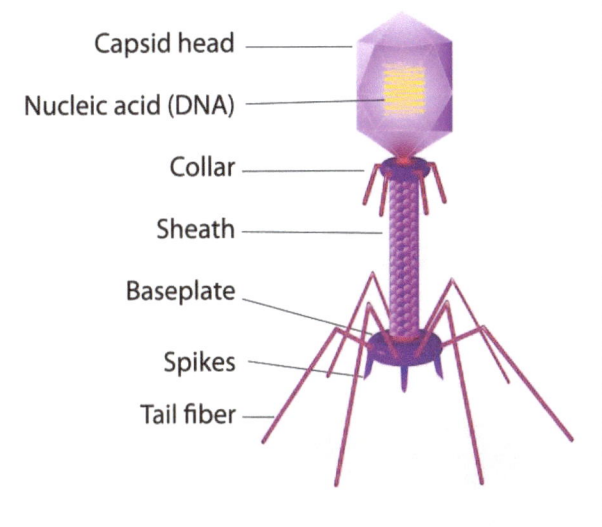
2. Tail: The tail is composed of a central hollow core which is cylindrical in shape surrounded by a contractile sheath (protein). It measures approx. 130 mm in length. The tail of phage T_4 is 100 nm in length and 25 nm in diameter.	Fig. 4. Bacteriophage structure
3. Terminal base plate with tail fibers (usually six in number).	
4. Spikes: Each corner of base plate contains a short pin or spike.	

Life Cycle of Bacteriophage and Replication of Viruses:

<u>Viruses</u> infect any type of living cells. It can be <u>animal cells</u>, <u>plant cells</u> and <u>bacterial cells</u>.

There are two viral replication strategies; when the virus kills the host cell it is called the **lytic cycle**, and when the virus does not kill the host but replicates when the host replicates it is called the **lysogenic cycle.**

Phages are usually specific for a few bacterial strains, because of the presence of phage specific receptors.

A. Lytic Cycle:

The replication cycle of virulent phage is divided into five sequential phases:
1. Adsorption,
2. Penetration,
3. Synthesis of phage components,
4. Maturation and assembly, and
5. Release of progeny viruses:

1. Adsorption:
The phage particles **attaches to a specific receptor site on the host cell membrane by means of tail fibers after** coming into contact by random collision. Adsorption occurs within minutes of contact.

2. Penetration:
After adsorption of phage to bacteria, the base plate and tail fibers of virus hold the bacterial cell firmly and the tail sheath of phage contracts. Phage muramidase present on the base plate weakened the part of cell wall. **T**he hollow core is pushed downwards through the weakened part of cell-wall to pass the viral nucleic acid.

The viral nucleic acid passes down the hollow tube into the host cell without penetrating into the cell wall. The empty head (capsid) and tail remains outside of the cell wall as shell or ghost.

3. Synthesis of phage components:
After the release of nucleic acid into the bacterial cell, the viral genome directs the biosynthetic machinery of host cell to produce components of new virus particles. This is affected by synthesis of specific enzymes (called early proteins) necessary for synthesis of phage components.

4. Maturation and assembly:
During maturation there is spontaneous assembly of phage protein in DNA- head and tail. Each component of phage nucleic acid acquires a protein coat. The tail structures are added forming a virion (infective virus particle).

5. Release:
Phage enzyme (Muramidase) acts on cell wall during replication and weakens it. It becomes easy for the progeny phages to rapidly release by the lysis of the infected bacterium. As a result the infected bacterium assumes a spherical shape. Muramidase concentration rises in the late stage of growth cycle causing lysis of cell with release of progeny phage.

Eclipse phase:

The time interval between the phage nucleic acid entered into the bacterial cell till the appearance of first infectious intra-cellular phage particle is called **"eclipse phase"**. Since viruses cannot be detected during this time period in the infected cell. The time interval between infection of host cell and sudden increase in viral load is called **"latent period"**. The duration of eclipse phase is about 15-30 minutes in phages.

B. Lysogenic Cycle:

In lysogenic cycle, the vegetative phage integrates with the host cell chromosomes and is converted into prophage without lysis of bacterial cell. The prophage may be converted into a virulent vegetative (lytic) phase spontaneously or by physical and chemical agents (UV rays, H_2O_2, nitrogen mustard).

"Prophage" is a latent bacteriophage retaining its DNA. Host bacteria carry prophage within them and don't lyse the bacteria is called "lysogenic bacteria". Bacteriophage that parasitizes a host bacterium without lysing it is called "temperate phage". Prophage may be lost during multiplication of lysogenic bacteria by means of excision. The excised prophage can infect other bacterial cells making the lysogenic.

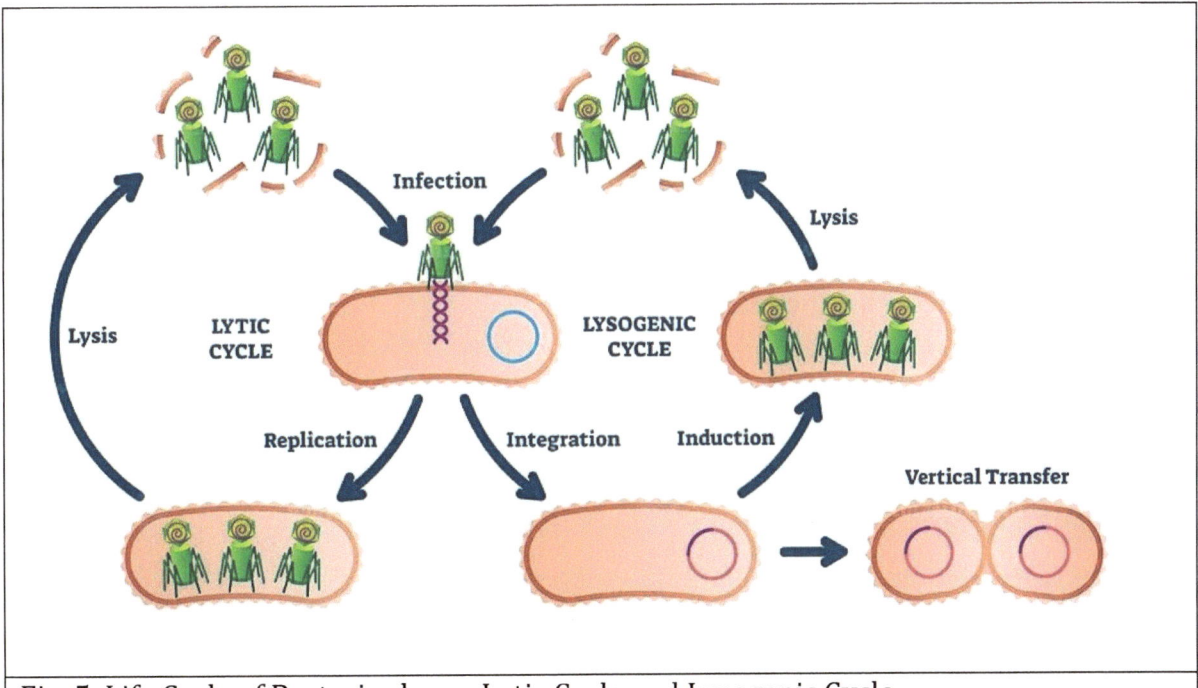

Fig. 5. Life Cycle of Bacteriophage- Lytic Cycle and Lysogenic Cycle

Significance of Bacteriophage:
1. **Phage Typing:** On the basis of the susceptibility of different strains of bacteria to different bacteriophages, the typing of bacteria can be done for identification and epidemiological studies.
2. **Phage Assay:** Phage plaque assay is used for tittering bacteriophage. After incubation, clear zones known as **plaques** are seen when phages grow on a lawn of susceptible strain culture of susceptible strain. These clear zones are known as **plaques.** A single phage produces only one plaque. Phage assay is a useful method in titrating the number of viable phages.
3. **Temperate Phage: They have an ability to choose between lytic or lysogenic life cycle. Hence,** Prophage genes may change the properties of host bacterium depending on either can integrate their genomes or replicates the phage genome. Such property of having chosen for selecting life cycle by bacteria following phage infection is called "**phage conversion**".
4. In transduction, genome is introduced by the virus in one bacterium cell to another, phages act as carriers of genes.
5. Phages can code for hundreds of monoclonal antibodies or genome following injection in bacterium in the cytoplasm. This makes them selective for use extensively in genetic engineering where they serve as cloning vectors.
6. They are responsible for natural removal of bacteria from water bodies

Morphology, Pathogenicity and Laboratory Diagnosis of Hepatitis Viruses

General Concepts

Viral hepatitis- includes hepatitis A, hepatitis B, and hepatitis C. They affect the liver and cause different hepatitis symptoms. Recreational drugs and prescription medications are other source of causes of hepatitis.

Hepatitis A virus

Morphology of Hepatitis A virus		Fig.6. Hepatitis A virus
Family	Picornaviridae;	
Genus	Hepatovirus	
Structure	Nonenveloped, icosahedral Nucleocapsid symmetry	
Shape	Spherical	
Size	27-32 nm in diameter	
Nucleic Acid	Single stranded RNA	

Mode of transmission: Fecal-oral route.

Incubation period: 10-50 days with a mode of ~1 month from exposure to symptoms regardless of the route of infection.

Pathogenicity:

1. Primary Disease Symptoms:
- Anicteric or icteric hepatitis
- Proteome of anorexia, fever (usually<39.5 C), fatigue, malaise, myalgia, nausea and vomiting, weight loss with disorder of taste and smell; right upper quadrat abdominal pain followed by an icteric phase within 10 days of the initial symptoms.

2. Severity of Clinical Disease:
Atypical manifestations include prolonged cholestasis, relapsing hepatitis, autoimmune chronic hepatitis, and extra hepatic manifestations (rash, arthritis, arthralgia, hemolytic anemia, pancreatitis, leukocytoclastic vasculitis, and renal disease).
Fulminant hepatitis (encephalopathy within 6-8 weeks of illness or 1-4 weeks after jaundice) is associated with high fever, marked abdominal pain, vomiting, and jaundice.

Screening and detection –
This test detects antibodies in the blood that are produced by the immune system in response to a hepatitis A infection.

At-Risk Populations:
- Unimmunized
- Native Americans
- Men who have sex with men
- Illegal drug users, injecting
- Persons with chronic liver disease (advanced fibrosis or cirrhosis)
- Persons and children's residing in areas where extended community outbreaks exist
- Refugees residing in temporary camps after catastrophes
- Children in day-care centers

Vector and Reservoir Involved:
- Infected humans and other primates

Prevention Measures:
- Routine vaccination of children.
- Vaccination of persons in groups at increased risk for hepatitis A or its adverse consequences and

• Using immune serum globulin for protection against hepatitis A administered to unvaccinated persons who are exposed to HAV within 2 weeks.

HEPATITIS B VIRUS:

Morphology of Hepatitis B virus		Hepatitis B virus
Family	Hepadnaviridae	
Genus	Orthohepadnavirus	
Structure	Icosahedral Nucleocapsid	
Shape	Spherical	
Size	• 42 nm in diameter (Dane particle- Virion) • 20 nm in diameter (Spherical Structures) • 22 nm in diameter (Filamentous Particles)	Fig.7. **Hepatitis B virus**
Nucleic Acid	Double-stranded DNA	
"HBsAg"	1. Outer shell (or envelope)	Composed of lipid and protein that is termed "surface antigen" or "HBsAg".
"HBcAg"	2. Core particle	Inner macromolecule protein shell that is known as the core particle or "HBcAg" contains the viral DNA and enzymes dedicated for viral replication (called "DNA polymerase").
"HBeAg"	3. Antigenic determinant	HBeAg (hepatitis B e antigen) is the antigenic determinant that is closely associated with the Nucleocapsid of HBV. It conjointly circulates as a soluble macromolecule protein in serum.

Epidemiology of Hepatitis B Virus:
- Worldwide, highest in sub-Saharan Africa and East Asia.

Mode of transmission:

- Contact with infectious (HBV) body fluids, such as blood, vaginal secretions, or semen.
- Use of Injection drug, having sex or sharing razors with an infected person.

Incubation period:
On average 75 days but may vary from 30-180 days.

Pathogenicity:
Acute and Chronic disease, conjointly related to primary carcinoma.
Only 30% to 50% of adults develop typical symptoms throughout acute infection.

- Fever, a flu-like illness, fatigue, dark urine, loss of appetite, nausea, vomiting, joint pain, clay-colored bowel movements, jaundice (yellowing of the skin and eyes), pain in the upper right abdomen (due to the inflamed liver).
- Hepatitis B virus causes serious liver conditions, such as liver cirrhosis or liver cancer.

Vector and Reservoir Involved:
- Humans and Mammals including woodchucks, beech ground squirrels and ducks.

Diagnosis of Hepatitis B
- The diagnosis of HBV infection and its associated disease is based on a combination of clinical, biochemical, histological, and serologic findings.
- **Immunoassay:** The laboratory can test for a wide range of HBV antigens and antibodies, using immunoassays based on enzyme reactivity (EIA) or chemiluminesence (CLIA) and ELISA.
- **PCR assay:** HBV DNA are often quantified in serum or plasma using real time polymerase chain reaction (PCR) assays.
- Detection of the Hepatitis B surface antigen, HBsAg.
- HBsAg and HBcAg indicate Acute HBV infection.
- Throughout the initial phase of infection, patients are also have detectable antibodies for hepatitis B e antigen (HBeAg) in the serum.
- HBeAg stands as a marker of high levels of virus load.
- HBsAg for at least 6 months indicates chronic infection. ButPersistent positive result for HBsAg is the principal marker of risk for developing chronic liver disease and liver cancer.

Prevention Measures
- Vaccination of infants as soon as possible after birth, preferably within 24 hours.
- Only disposable needles should be used

• Simple environmental procedures will limit the chances of infection to health care employees, laboratory personnel, and others.

Vaccines of Hepatitis B
- A vaccine for hepatitis B has been available since 1982.
- The Hepatitis B vaccine is safe and effective and is typically given as 3-4 shots over a 6-month period.
  1. Plasma-derived vaccines
  2. Recombinant DNA-derived vaccines
- The HBsAg vaccines (HB) can be combined with other vaccines such as Calmette-Guérin bacillus (BCG), measles, mumps, and rubella (MMR), Haemophilus influenza b (Hib), and diphtheria, tetanus and pertussis combined with polio (DTP-polio).

HEPATITIS C VIRUS:

Morphology of Hepatitis C virus	
Family	flaviviruses
Genus	Hepacivirus
Structure	Enveloped
Shape	Icosahedral
Size	Approx 60 nm in diameter
Nucleic Acid	Single-stranded RNA
Viral envelope	Two viral envelopeglycoproteins, E1 and E2, are embedded in the lipidenvelope.

Fig.8. **Hepatitis C virus**

Mode of transmission:
The hepatitis C virus is a blood borne virus. It is most commonly transmitted through:
- Sharing of injection for drug or else;
- The reuse or inadequate sterilization of medical equipment.
- The transfusion of HCV infected blood and blood products while transfusion.
- Transmitted sexually
- From infected mother to her baby in her womb.

Epidemiology: Worldwide. The most affected regions are WHO Eastern Mediterranean and European Regions.

Incubation period:
2 weeks to 6 months

Pathogenicity:
Those who are acutely symptomatic may exhibit fever, fatigue, decreased appetite, nausea, vomiting, abdominal pain, dark urine, grey-colored feces, joint pain and jaundice (yellowing of skin and the whites of the eyes).

Screening and diagnosis
The infection remains asymptomic and often goes undiagnosed until decades. The secondary symptoms develop by that point serious liver injury happens.

HCV infection is diagnosed by following steps:
1. Screening test for anti-HCV antibodies with a serological test. About 15–45% of individuals infected with HCV spontaneously clear the infection by a robust immunological response without the requirement for treatment. Although no longer infected, they will still test positive for anti-HCV antibodies.
2. A nucleic acid test for HCV ribonucleic acid (RNA) for confirmation of chronic infection is done.
3. Liver biopsy, for an assessment of the degree of liver damage (fibrosis and cirrhosis). This can be done by liver biopsy or through a variety of non-invasive tests.
   For treatment decisions and management of the disease following guide are considered
   - The degree of liver damage and
   - Virus genotype

At-Risk Populations:
- Drug adductors, uses injections and intranasal drugs;
- Recipients of infected blood products.
- Children born to mothers infected with HCV;
- Having sex with HCV-infected and or HIV infected partner;
- Prisoners or previously incarcerated persons; and
- People who totattoos or piercings.

Host Involved: Humans

Prevention Measures:
- Hand hygiene: including surgical hand preparation, hand washing and use of gloves;
- Provision of comprehensive harm-reduction services to people who inject drugs including sterile injecting equipment;
- Screening of donated blood for hepatitis B and C before blood transfusion;
- Training of health personnel; and
- Consistent use of condoms.

HEPATITIS D VIRUS:

Morphology of Hepatitis D virus		Fig. 9.Hepatitis D virus
Family	Unassigned	
Genus	*Delta virus*	
Structure	Single-stranded, circular	
Shape	Spherical	
Size	36 nm diameter	
Nucleic Acid	RNA	
HDAg	Produce one protein, namely HDAg.	
HDAg-S	Produced in the early stages of an infection	
HDAg-L	Produced in the later stages of an infection.	

Mode of transmission:

The infection is contagious and spread through direct contact with -
- Vaginal fluids
- Semen
- Blood
- Birth (from mother to her newborn)

Also by sharing syringes and receiving clotting factor concentrates infected with HDV.

Epidemiology:

HDV is common in the immediate Mediterranean region, sub-Saharan Africa, the Middle East, and the northern part of South America.

Incubation period:
- Co-infection is 90 days (range 45-160 days)
- Super infection is approximately 2-8 weeks.

Pathogenicity:

Acute hepatitis: infection with HBV and HDV can lead to a mild-to-severe or even fulminant hepatitis. The recovery is usually complete with proper treatment and medication. The development of chronic hepatitis D is rare.

Super infection: The super infection of HDV on chronic hepatitis B accelerates progression to cirrhosis and a more severe disease.

Symptoms:

Hepatitis D doesn't always cause symptoms. When symptoms do occur, they usually include:
- Yellowing of the skin and eyes, which is called jaundice
- Joint pain
- Abdominal pain
- Vomiting
- Loss of appetite
- Dark urine
- Fatigue

The symptoms of hepatitis B and hepatitis D are so similar that it becomes difficult to determine the causative agent. In some cases, hepatitis D will make the symptoms of hepatitis B worse. It can even cause symptoms in people who have hepatitis B but who never had symptoms.

Screening and diagnosis
1. High titers of Immunoglobulin G (IgG) and Immunoglobulin M (IgM) anti-HDV give the diagnosis of HDV infection.
2. Detection of HDV RNA in serum confirms the diagnosis.
3. HDV diagnostics are not widely available.
4. There is no standardization for HDV RNA assays.

At-Risk Populations:
- Injection drug users
- Persons with hemophilia
- Infants/children of immigrants from areas with high rates of HBV infection
- Household contacts of chronically infected persons
- Persons with multiple sex partners or diagnosis of a sexually transmitted disease
- Men who have sex with men
- Sexual contacts of infected persons
- Infants born to infected mothers
- Health care and public safety workers
- Hemodialysis patients

Host Involved: Humans

Prevention Measures: Vaccination

HEPATITIS E VIRUS:

Morphology of Hepatitis E virus	
Family	Hepeviridae
Genus	Hepevirus
Structure	Nonenveloped, icosahedral Nucleocapsid symmetry
Shape	Spherical
Size	30-34 nm diameter
Nucleic Acid	Single stranded RNA

Fig. 10. **Hepatitis E virus**

Mode of transmission:
- Commonly- fecal-oral,
- Person-to-person spread relatively uncommon and
- Blood transmission is rare.

Epidemiology: world-wide.

In regions of the world where sanitation may be poor (Asia, Africa and Central America). Historically hepatitis E was considered a travel-associated infection, and the disease may have been under diagnosed.

Incubation period: Usually 3-8 weeks

Pathogenicity and Symptoms:
Usually the infection is self-limiting and resolves within 2–6 weeks. Fulminant hepatitis (acute liver failure) could be a serious disease that happens terribly seldom.

Typical signs and symptoms of hepatitis include:
- Mild fever, anorexia, nausea and vomiting; some persons may also have abdominal pain, itching (without skin lesions), skin rash, or joint pain.
- Jaundice (yellow discoloration of the skin and sclera of the eyes), with dark urine and pale stools; and
- A slightly enlarged and tender liver (hepatomegaly).

In immunocompromised patients—particularly in solid organ transplanted patients—hepatitis E may cause a chronic infection.

Screening and diagnosis

1. IgG and IgM antibody assays have been developed but vary widely in sensitivity and specificity.
2. Virus detected by RT-PCR.
3. A confirmed acute case is defined as either a PCR positive or IgM and IgG positive.

At-Risk Populations:
- Endemic and epidemic in residents of Southeast and Central Asia plus Japan, Middle East, North and West Africa, Mexico, Brazil
- Travelers to these areas
- Sporadic cases occur in developed nations.

Host Involved:
Humans

Prevention Measures:
- Cooking meat and meat products thoroughly.
- Avoid eating raw or undercooked meat and shellfish
- Hand Hygiene before preparing, serving and eating food
- Ensuring a clean drinking water even when travelling.

Morphology, Pathogenicity and Laboratory Diagnosis of HIV / AIDS Virus.

Family	Retroviridae
Genus	Lentivirus
Shape	Cone-shaped
Nucleic Acid	RNA
Nucleocapsid	Composed of the core protein p24.
Structure	Icosahedral
Size	100 nm in diameter
External spikes	72
Envelope	Two major envelope glycoproteins gp120 and gp41.
Types of the AIDS virus	HIV-1 and HIV-2

Structure of HIV / AIDS

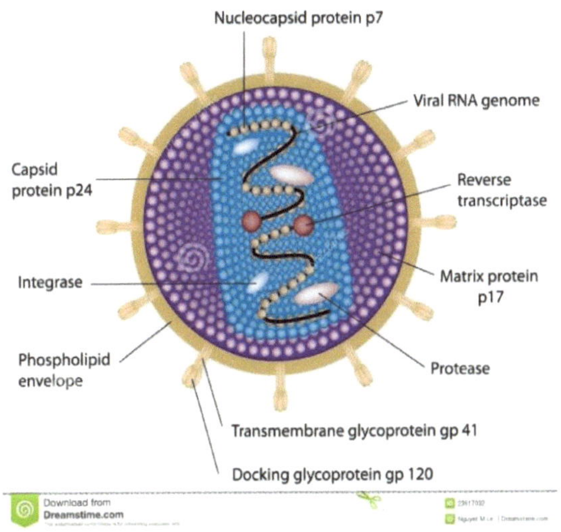

Fig.11. **Structure of HIV / AIDS**

Human Immunodeficiency Virus (HIV) key features-

The major serological differences reside in the surface protein gp120.	
Subtypes or 'clades'	HIV-1 and HIV-2 are further separated into subtypes or 'clades' due to the variable gp120 protein.
Nucleocapsid	HIV has a characteristic dense, cone-shaped Nucleocapsid composed of the core protein p24. This has two identical copies of single-stranded RNA genome which are associated with the viral enzymes.
Viral enzymes	Reverse transcriptase (RT), RNase H, integrase and protease.

HIV encodes 3 structural genes and 6 regulative genes.

	Structural genes:	
1. Group Specific Antigen (Gag):	p24, p7, p17)	
2. Envelope (Env):	gp 120, gp 41	
	a.	On the basis of gp120 genes HIV is divided into subtypes (clades): A through I
	b.	gp120 binds to CD4 on CD4+ T lymphocytes and cells of the monocyte/macrophage lineage and co receptors (CCR5 and CXCR4)
	c.	gp41 mediate fusion between the cellular and viral membranes.
3. Polymerase (Pol):	Reverse transcriptase, integrase, protease	

Regulatory genes found in HIV	
Required for replication	
1. Tat:	Activation of transcription of viral genes
2. Rev:	Transport of late mRNAs from nucleus to cytoplasm
Not required for replication	
1. Nef (negative factor) protein:	Decreases CD4 and MHC class I protein expression in virus infected cells (mutation in the nef gene).
2. Vif:	Enhances viral infectivity
3. Vpr:	Transports viral core from cytoplasm into nucleus
4. Vpu:	Enhances virion release from cell.

Mode of transmission:

The HIV virus is often transmitted via unprotected sexual activity, blood transfusions, hypodermic needles, and from mother to child.

Pathophysiology of HIV:

Upon acquisition of the virus, the virus replicates within and kills T helper cells that are required for nearly all adaptive immune responses. It is associated with initial period of illness which often misleads the particular and significant diagnosis and later becomes asymptomatic. When the CD4 lymphocyte count falls below 200 cells/ml of blood, the HIV host has progressed to AIDS, a condition characterized by deficiency in cell-mediated immunity and the resulting increased susceptibility to opportunistic infections and certain forms of cancer.

HIV infection passes through a series of steps or stages before it turns into AIDS. These stages of infection are outlined in 1993 by the Centers for Disease Control and prevention is:

1. **Seroconversion illness** – this occurs in 1 to 6 weeks after acquiring the infection. The feeling is similar to as of respiratory illness like flu.
2. **Asymptomatic infection** – Virus levels are low and replication continues slowly. CD4 and CD8 lymphocyte levels are normal. This stage has no symptoms and may persist for years together.
3. **Persistent generalized lymphadenopathy (PGL)** – The swollen of lymph nodes in these patients for three months or longer.
4. **Symptomatic infection** – This stage manifests with symptoms in the infected patient. In addition, there may be opportunistic infections in immunocompromised patients.
5. **AIDS** – this stage is characterised by severe immunodeficiency. There are signs of life-threatening infections and unusual tumors. This stage is characterized by CD4 T-cell count below 200 cells/mm^3.

Laboratory diagnosis of HIV Infection-

Sample Collection and Transport
- Whole blood (10 mL) is sufficient.
- Specimens can be stored at room temperature up to 3 days, at 4°C for up to 7 days.
- The serum or plasma must be separated from the clot or cells and stored at -20°C for longer storage.
- Specimens for PCR are considered as STAT. These samples must be processed within 48 hours of collection.

Virus cultivation

Virus can be isolated from infected persons in most phases of the infection.
A positive result is recognized by either ways-

1. Appearance of virus antigen (p 24) or
2. Reverse transcriptase activity in the culture medium.

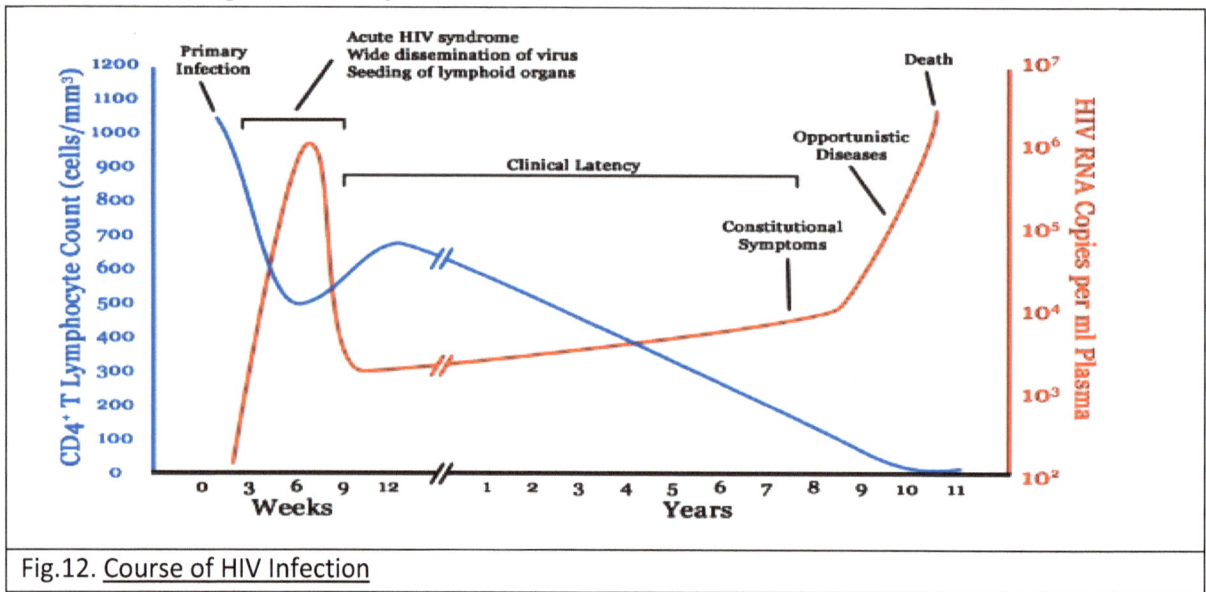

Fig.12. Course of HIV Infection

Antigen/Antibody detection

Antibodies usually become detectable from 3 to 12 weeks after infection. An infected person remains positive for antibody for life, but titers often fall in patients with AIDS.

Indirect and competitive ELISA is mostly considered best choice as the technique can also use as mixture of viral antigens. It is recommended that confirmatory tests ELISA tests or Western blot; to exclude the possibility of false positive results.

1. Point of Care tests (POCT) for HIV

these tests offers rapid, on-site HIV screening test leads to a format that's comparatively straightforward to perform.

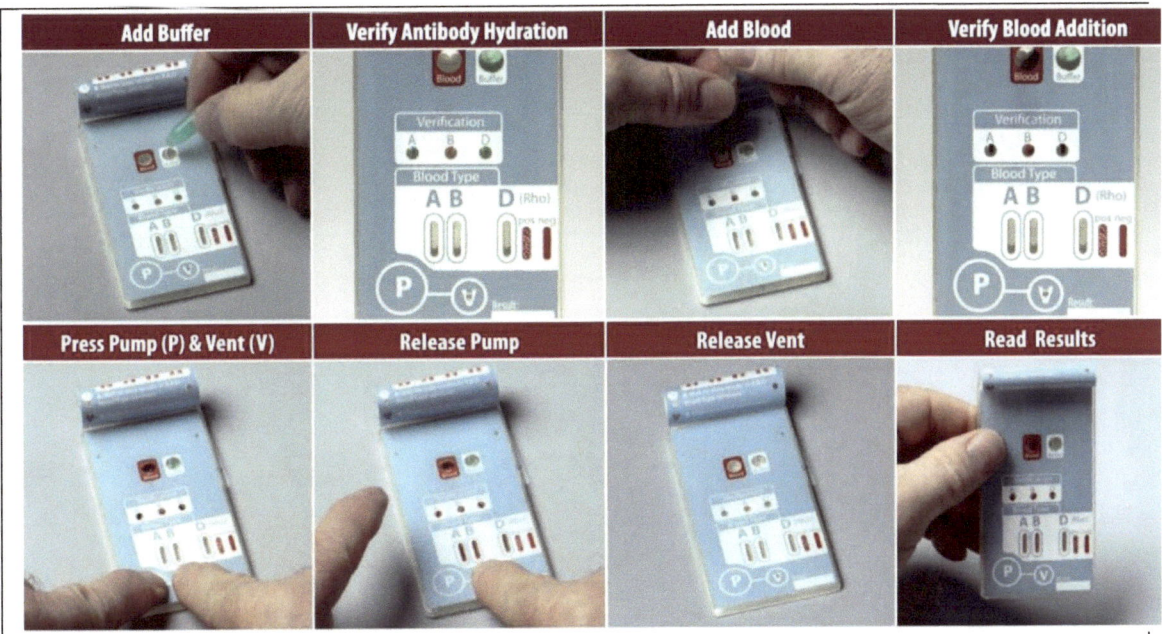
Fig.13. POCT steps for HIV

2. **ELISA for HIV diagnosis**

   it is a commonly used as a screening assay for HIV. It is highly sensitive test but false positives can be seen. Current 'window period' (the time from exposure to Seroconversion) for HIV is less than 3 weeks in most cases.

3. **p24 antigen testing**

   p24 antigen tests are also enzyme immuno-assay (EIA) based.

   P24 antigen test is useful
   - For specimens from patients that are high risk and symptomatic but HIV EIA-negative (for Ab testing), or
   - For specimens that are EIA-positive but Western blot-negative or – indeterminate
   - For confirmation of neonatal HIV infection

4. **Viral genome amplification (PCR)**

The PCR technique amplify target HIV-DNA present in minute amounts and makes is more sensitive and specific method for the diagnosis of HIV infection. It PCR application are as follows-
- Within the identification of HIV infection in infants born to infected mothers.
- Resolving indeterminate Western blot results and
- Testing immune compromised individuals who may not mount an antibody response.

- Quantitative determination of virion RNA by reverse transcription PCR (RT-PCR) to follow progression of HIV infection in untreated patients and to monitor the effects of antiviral chemotherapy in patients. It is used in conjunction with CD4 counts.

5. **Western blot Test**

    Western blot immune blot is a highly specific diagnosis of HIV infection. This allows for the visual interpretation of antibodies to the corresponding structural polypeptides of HIV.

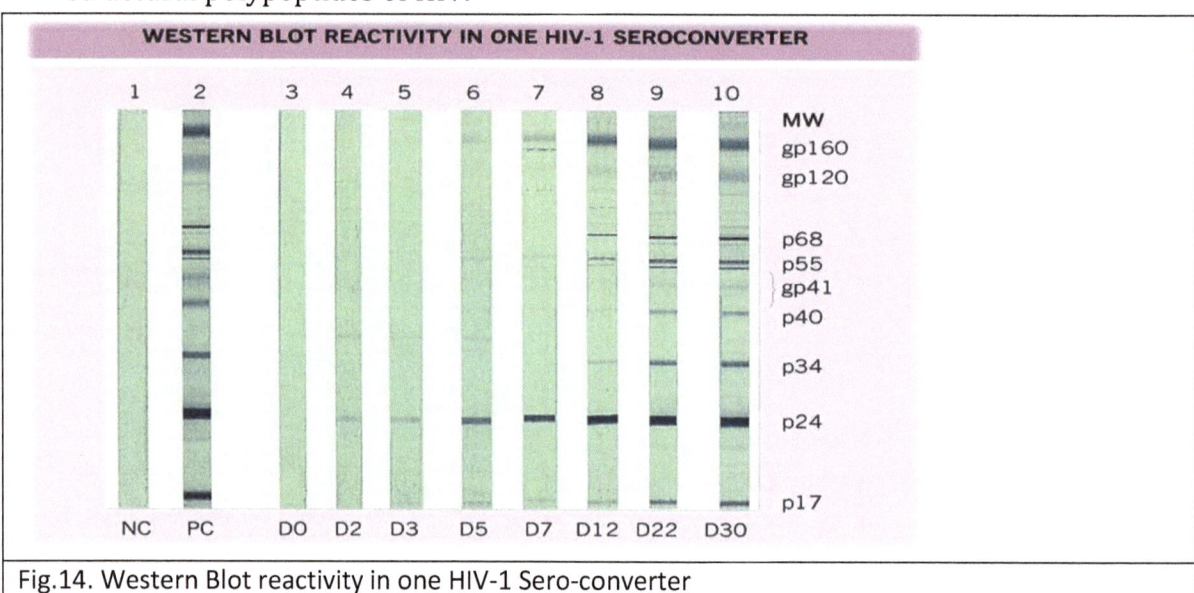

Fig.14. Western Blot reactivity in one HIV-1 Sero-converter

6. **CD4+ lymphocyte count**

The depletion of CD4+ lymphocytes is the hallmark of chronic HIV infection. Therefore monitoring of CD4+ lymphocyte count is an important determinant for clinical staging, initiation of antiviral therapy and *Pneumocystis jiroveci* pneumonia prophylaxis.

7. **NATs:** It is the most accurate for recent exposure and hence is used to detect HIV between 7 and 28 days. But the test is extremely expensive.

Oncogenic viruses.

During the viral replication process, genome affects the host cell's genes in such a ways that it may cause it to become cancerous. These viruses are referred to as oncogenic viruses, which means viruses that cause or give rise to tumors.

VIRUS	Disease	CANCER
Papovaviridae Papillomavirus (some)	Warts, including STD genital warts	Uterine (Cervical) cancer
Herpesviridae Lymphocryptovirus (Epstein-Barr virus)	Infectious mononucleosis	Burkitt's lymphoma nasopharyngeal carcinoma Hodgkin's disease
Hepadnavirus Hepatitis B virus (HBV)	Hepatitis B virus (infectious hepatitis)	Liver cancer
Adenoviridae	Acute respiratory disease; Common cold	Adenocarcinomas (Cancer of glandular epithelial tissues)
Poxviridae	Smallpox; cowpox	Miscellaneous

Oncogenic RNA Viruses of the family Retro-viridae	
VIRUS	CANCER
Human T-cell leukemia virus (HTLV-1; HTLV-2)	Lymphoma
Sarcoma viruses of cats, chickens, rodents	Sarcomas (cancer of connective tissues)
Mammary tumor virus of mice	Mammary gland tumors
Feline leukemia virus (FeLV)	Feline leukemia

REFERENCES

http://cnx.org/contents/tK8Muj08@12/Viruses
https://www.microrao.com/micronotes/bacteriophage.pdf
https://www.ncbi.nlm.nih.gov/books/NBK7864/
https://www.aabb.org/tm/eid/Documents/87s.pdf
http://www.who.int/mediacentre/factsheets/fs164/en/
http://www.health.state.mn.us/divs/idepc/diseases/hepatitis/hepdfact.pdf
https://www.aabb.org/tm/eid/Documents/93s.pdf
https://www.gov.uk/government/publications/hepatitis-e-symptoms-transmission-prevention-treatment/hepatitis-e-symptoms-transmission-treatment-and-prevention
http://www.who.int/mediacentre/factsheets/fs280/en/
https://microbeonline.com/laboratory-diagnosis-of-hiv-virus/
https://en.wikipedia.org/wiki/Pathophysiology_of_HIV/AIDS
https://www.cdc.gov/hepatitis/hbv/bfaq.htm
www.biologydiscussion.com/viruses/...latent period
https://en.wikipedia.org/wiki/Pathophysiology_of_HIV/AIDS - Pathophysiology of HIV
https://en.wikipedia.org/wiki/Virus_classification - LHT System of Virus Classification
https://books.google.ae/books?isbn=9350255103 - The head of phage T4 has a diameter of 65 nm and is 100 nm long.
https://microbiologyinfo.com › Diseases - Hepatitis B virusNucleic Acid
- https://wellonapharma.wordpress.com/tag/hepatitis/- Symptoms:Hepatitis D
/www.virology.ws/tag/chorioallantoic-membrane
https://microbiologyinfo.com › Basic Microbiology
https://microbiologyinfo.com› Basic Microbiology
https://academic.oup.com/cid/article/31/3/739/297506
https://www.coursehero.com › Washington University in St. Louis › L41 › L41 349
https://norkinvirology.wordpress.com/.../felix-dherelle-the-discovery-of-bacteriophag
https://books.google.ae/books?isbn=9350255103
www.biologydiscussion.com/viruses/bacteriophage-introduction...and-life.../31035
www.biologydiscussion.com/viruses/bacteriophage-introduction
https://en.wikipedia.org/wiki/Bacteriophage
www.biologydiscussion.com/viruses/bacteriophage-introduction
https://www.sciencedirect.com/topics/immunology-and-microbiology/phage-typing
www.scnow.com/living/article_54bcc88a-f798-11e6-9ef7-bf50088a49f5.html
https://en.wikipedia.org/wiki/North_Africa
https://www.medicinenet.com/nausea_and_vomiting/article.htm1
https://en.wikipedia.org/wiki/Structure_and_genome_of_HIV
www.catie.ca/en/pif/fall-2011/recently-infected-individuals-priority-hiv-prevention
...https://www.omicsonline.org/.../acquired-immuno-deficiency-syndrome-peer-reviewe
...?www.thebodypro.com/content/48385/hiv-testing-basic-questions-and-answers.html

Figure	Reference
1.	https://www.dreamstime.com/stock-illustration-icosahedron-gold-three-dimensional-shape-platonic-solid-geometry-polyhedron-twenty-triangular-faces-thirty-edges-image41363107
2.	https://www.easynotecards.com/print_list/68884
3.	https://www.google.com/search?q=chick+embryo+inoculation+free+for+commercial+use&tbm=isch&ved=2ahUKEwi1-e_y9Y_qAhXKwIUKHd8bBm8Q2-
4.	*https://www.dreamstime.com/stock-images-structure-virus-bacteriophage-image27111334*
5.	https://istudy.pk/bacterial-transduction/
6.	https://www.liverdoctor.com/liver-problems/hepatitis/
7.	https://en.wikipedia.org/wiki/Hepatitis_B_virus
8.	https://en.wikipedia.org/wiki/Hepatitis_C_virus
9.	https://en.wikipedia.org/wiki/Hepatitis_D
10.	http://www.jotscroll.com/forums/11/posts/91/hepatitis-e-symptoms-vaccine-diagnosis-treatment.html
11.	https://www.dreamstime.com/stock-photography-structure-hiv-image23617032
12.	https://www.researchgate.net/figure/A-generalized-graph-of-the-relationship-between-HIV-copies-viral-load-and-CD4-counts_fig1_242611621
13.	http://www.mdpi.com/2079-6374/5/3/577htm
14.	https://microbeonline.com/western-blot-technique-principle-procedures-advantages-and-disadvantages/

www.ingramcontent.com/pod-product-compliance
Lightning Source LLC
Chambersburg PA
CBHW041939240526

45473CB00037B/2270